<u>Communica</u>

<u>Relationship</u>

The Definitive Guide To Overcome Couple Conflicts And Anxiety If You Feel Insecure In Love, Acquiring Powerful Communication Skills and Techniques for a Happier Relationship

Table of Contents:

DR. RACHEL R. MILLER

Introduction

Communication is an essential pillar of a successful relationship. You should be open and honest with your partner and let them know what you're thinking. Communication in your relationship is super important. It's the key to a healthy relationship. Being able to communicate effectively with your partner can make or break your relationship. A good relationship is built on trust plus understanding. Communication is the key ingredient in building trust and understanding. If something is bothering you, you need to let your partner know what is going on. If you don't communicate your feelings, you'll never know if something is bothering them. Communication is your solution to a healthy relationship with your partner.

Communication plays an essential role in a relationship. Studies have shown that couples who communicate problems and conflicts with each other are healthier and more satisfied with their marriages than those who do not. Studies show that couples who can talk openly about their problems live happier lives and have better sex lives than those who experience communication breakdowns. Communication can help you resolve conflicts and understand each other's needs.

In a healthy relationship, communication is how two people express their feelings and work together to solve problems. Communication can also be used to set rules or boundaries for the couple. There are many different forms of communication. You use verbal communication by talking to each other. Verbal communication can include expressing your thoughts and feelings verbally, sharing ideas, asking your partner questions, and telling them about your day or experiences. Nonverbal communication is another way to communicate with each other. It involves using gestures, actions, and facial expressions to get your point across. These two will also be tackles throughout this guide.

Without it, relationships can suffer and become strained. Communication indeed is a very vital skill for having a successful relationship. Communication is a two-way method that requires both people to participate when they interact with each other actively. Effective communication is an excellent problem-solver and one of the best ways to deal with all aspects of your relationship effectively. The longer you know your mate, the more you understand how they react in different situations. But don't assume how your mate feels unless he or she has said so.

The successful way to make good communication is by improving your listening skill. You should have your full attention on what your partner says to you. If you want to listen, you need to be willing to listen actively and give it some focus and time. Don't let anything distracts your attention. You need to hear not only what people say but also what's behind the words they say. And pay attention to both mind and heart. That's how you can listen to your partner and make good communication with them.

Some couples indeed have a difficult time communicating, but it is possible to improve your communication significantly. Communication is an art and takes lots of practice and willpower. However, if both partners are willing to try and try, it can make a huge difference in the relationship. You may not be perfect initially, but with your efforts, you will see how much better communication can help you understand each other better than before. With this ultimate guide in your hand, we believe you will improve your communication with your partner. So let's start!

Chapter 1- Talking About Difficult Topics

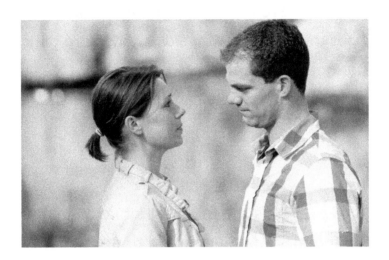

There will be some tough situations and difficult topics that will be brought up in any relationship. These heavy conversations aren't often happily anticipated, but they are necessary. We will go over what these conversations could be, tips on handling and addressing them, and why we should not avoid these important but difficult conversations.

Difficult Topics Many People Have to Face During Their Relationships

There is a wide variety of topics that people find difficult in their daily lives and relationships, which is different for everyone. However, we're going to highlight some of the most difficult roadblocks people come upon in their relationships so you can get an idea of the types of difficult topics we're referring to in my advice throughout this part. As we said, many more difficult topics are not covered here, but the ones we've listed are ones that many people can relate to across the board.

Loss

The loss of a loved is the toughest situation in anyone's life. Therefore, it can be very hard to talk about. The key here is to consider your partner if they are going through loss and be there to support them. It can be not easy to know what to say in these situations, and sometimes silence is best, but try to let your partner know how much you care about them and that you are there whenever they need you. Discussing feelings after a loss can be hard, but it is a big part of the overall healing process.

Sexual Consent

Sexual consent is one of the more awkward topics we talk about in our relationships. Still, we all must discuss our health, emotional wellbeing, and the stability of our relationships. Sexual consent conversations include but are not limited to: the use of protection and contraceptives, discussions about STI disclosure, the desire for whether or not to have children, the limits of sex positions, bondage, hard limits, exclusivity, and more. These discussions must take place for your safety and comfort in sexual situations to have a good relationship.

In-Laws

If you are married, in-laws are going to come into the picture. It can be challenging at times because you may feel like you are coming between your spouse and their family, or you may feel as though they are struggling to choose between you or their family. This power struggle between you and your spouse's family can put a big strain on your relationship and discussing your anxieties about this may seem overwhelming. Don't fear your partner's reaction during these conversations and try to be as open and honest as you can be without pointedly attacking their family. It's a fine line that is hard to learn to walk, but if you discuss your in-laws with your spouse openly, it will turn out all right.

Betrayal

We don't like to think it will happen to us, but betrayal can sometimes occur in a relationship. When this happens, your partner's trust is fragile, you start questioning the relationship, and negative emotions start to stir. It can be challenging to talk about this topic with your partner because you may feel incredibly hurt and angry, but you have to if you want to mend the relationship. If your partner has betrayed your trust and no longer wishes to be with them, that is your call, but it is always a good idea to talk it out first and gain closure about the situation. Your emotions in this instant are entirely valid but be the better person and hear what they have to say.

Money Problems

Money problems happen; it's just a natural speed bump in life. When they happen, however, you may feel stressed, embarrassed, and several other negative emotions. Instead of pushing those feelings away to hide your embarrassment from your partner, it is a good idea to reach out to them for support during that difficult time. They will likely be able to walk you through your issues and help you through your struggles. As a team, it's always best to work these things through together. Don't let your fear of embarrassment, tension, or argument keep you from being truthful about your finances or feelings.

Sickness and Other Health Issues

If you hide your health issues from your partner, it will hurt your health, fracture the relationship's trust, and make it impossible for your partner to help you through it and support you. I know sickness and health problems can be scary, but that is what your partner is there for! If you are in it for the long-run, you will want them to know what is ailing you so they can help you every step of the way. You are not a burden to them, and if they truly care, they will want to make sure you are ok above all else.

Past Relationships

Ok, this is a big one. Most people do not want to bring up their past relationships because it can be very embarrassing, emotional, and awkward. It may also make your partner feel as though you are comparing them to an ex. Sometimes, however, it is important to discuss your past with your partner to understand if certain insecurities pop up. If you discuss those insecurities with your partner, then if something makes you uncomfortable, they will know it is not because of them but because of a traumatic experience in your past. Open up to your partner in the right way, and it will strengthen your bond. You can talk about past abusive relationships, distrustful ones, triggers, and the like, but here are some things that should be avoided for the health of your relationship: sex life, pet peeves, physical features, favorite date spots, songs that remind you of an ex, etc. It is good to talk about exes in some regards; make sure to tread lightly and be smart about it.

How to Handle Difficult Conversations

Problem Solve and Tackle it Like a Team

The most important tip we can give you is to handle difficult situations as a team. If you try to be right all the time or figure things out together, it can make your partner feel useless or like they are not a true part of the team. Work together to tackle these difficult topics so you can overcome things as a unit and grow together. It will strengthen your relational bonds, make it easier to tackle similar situations in the future and prevent your relationship from slowly fracturing over time. Remember, it's all about fixing the issue at hand and not one-upping your partner, especially in sensitive situations. Don't offer unwarranted advice or negate the comments that your partner makes. Instead, lean on one another and fight every battle as a team.

Be Positive

It is very important to remain positive during a difficult situation. If you start making negative comments or retreating from an issue, it can cause stress, frustration, sadness, depression, and more that will cause the situation to spiral out of control. Take a deep breath, keep a level head, and try to be optimistic about the outcome of any situation you may have to face with your partner. In the end, if you want the situation to turn out ok, you have to believe that it will be so. Use compassion, smile, let yourself believe that things will get better, and lean on your partner. You can get through this; you have to try! Express gratitude at the strength the both of you have for even bringing up the topic and admire each other's courage. Thank one another for their courage, even. Pep yourself and your partner up and be strong, and you will know that you can tackle anything the world can throw at the two of you!

Don't Put Your Walls Up

Shutting down during difficult conversations and putting your walls up makes it very difficult for your partner to reach your level, understand what is going on, and help you tackle it. It can make it ten times harder to overcome adversity, and it is not healthy for you, your partner, or your relationship. Trust your partner and let your walls down. Express those emotions you are trying to hide and work through every situation together. You don't have to do this alone. That is what partnership is all about. You have to be trusting and vulnerable so you can navigate those difficult waters together. Be open and honest with these difficult subjects, making all of the smaller things so much easier. If you can open up to your partner and get through the hardest relationship conversations together, you can do anything! What is there to fear?

Utilize Empathy

Empathy and compassion are imperative during difficult situations. If things are rocky, it makes it a lot easier to navigate the situation if you are both open to seeing one another's perspectives and emotions so that you know how to tread carefully. Listen intently to your partner's words during difficult conversations because you know it must have been hard for them to bring it up in the first place, and they care about you enough to open up and trust you with the situation. Understanding this part is the first step to take. Then, make sure you give your full attention and remain invested throughout the entire conversation. Don't check out just because the conversation makes you uncomfortable or embarrassed. If your partner trusts you enough to bring the subject up, it is important enough for you to at least listen and offer support. Discuss the issue with your heart and lovingly find a solution together.

Give it All the Time it Needs

Don't skimp and speed through difficult conversations just because it feels uncomfortable. It is degrading the topic's importance, and it can make your partner feel that you are disinterested and uncaring about the situation. Additionally, choose the time for you to approach your partner wisely. Don't bombard your partner with it right as they walk through the door to get it out of the way. Choose a calm, stable time to discuss difficult topics to make sure that you are both on level ground. If you do it during an abrupt or busy time of day, the issue will not be resolved conclusively, and you will be right back to square one. Make sure to discuss this with your partner and ensure that you are both good enough to start a conversation regarding the subject. Ask your partner or spouse, "Is this a good time to talk?" "Can we discuss something that has been on my mind?" "Are you feeling well enough to discuss something important right now?" "I need some help. Do you have a minute for us to sit and talk?" and "When would you be comfortable discussing this issue?" to feel out the environment and pick the best time.

Chapter 2- Avoid Fighting/Arguing

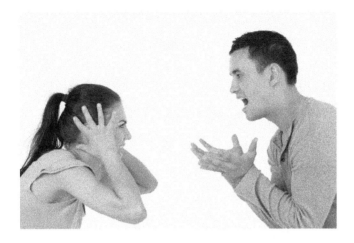

Fighting is almost a natural occurrence in a relationship because it is bound to happen if your partner does something that does not please you. However, this is not a reason to make everything worse because there is always a way you can get around the problems that affect you.

One such way is to avoid suppressing problems from the past and bringing them out when you argue with your partner. It is not a good thing to bring up issues from the past because it shows that you have a problem letting go and can easily affect your relationship.

When your partner wrongs or blame you in any way, discuss it immediately and get it through with. Arguments thrive when the partner constantly brings up the mistakes you probably apologized for, which frustrates the relationship to inevitable failure.

Similarly, do not let your anger be locked up inside you for an excessive amount of time. You might be sitting with your partner happy, but you are completely upset with them deep within. Let them know that you are not pleased with something they did, do not keep it within you for a long time.

The disadvantage of stockpiling your anger is that you will almost be uncontrollable when you argue with your partner. They will not be aware of you being angry with them at an unusual time because of an already passed issue.

When you become angry, your body reacts in a specific way that can put you very much at ease. As small as it might seem, it is important to pay attention to how your body reacts because it results from the release of chemicals and inflames your feelings.

It is necessary to calm down because you can always speak in a controlled way with your partner without affecting them adversely. Being calm and positioned will eliminate the chances of arguing with them and settling any issues you have with them reasonably.

If you wish to stop fighting with your partner, then stop raising your voice whenever you argue. It will surprise you just how calming it is to be calm and minimize the noise you cause whenever you are arguing with them.

Speak calmly no matter how grave the problem is, and the chances are that you will find a way past it. Nobody likes arguing, particularly with somebody you love so much. So the solution is to whisper, and it will surprisingly change the dimensions of how you communicate with your partner.

When you argue with your partner, consider that there is a difference between rage and anger. When you are angry, you can state your feelings and focus on finding a solution to your problems. It is possible to calm yourself down, particularly if your partner is reasonable with you.

However, when you are enraged, you can threaten your partner's relationship, and only after you have broken up will you realize your mistake. It is necessary to control your feelings because your partner is your better half and can come up with solutions that will benefit both of you.

It is possible to avoid an argument by simply not arguing. If your partner is trying to goad you into an argument, avoid it and pretend like you are not having a conversation in the first place. There is never any need to start a fight with somebody you love because you can always talk reasonably.

Arguments between couples are intriguing because both of you still care about each other. It is better to resolve the problem by having a calm conversation, and you will be surprised that you will start laughing with each other when you choose not to engage in an argument.

Before you choose to get angry at your partner, talk about your feelings, and let them know that something is upsetting you. It is possible to avoid an argument by bringing your anger into check. Let your partner know how you feel before launching an argument with them.

Communicating your feelings is the surest way of solving the dispute with your partner in a quick a reasonable manner. If your partner understands how you feel simply by verbalizing something they were not aware of, you have a better chance of communicating well with him.

It is also possible for you to sit down with your partner when your spirits are high and develop a problem-solving method for both of you. You can solve problems by having a conversation in a specific place that makes both of you calm.

You can also decide on a scheme where you get past problems by engaging in an activity of similar interest. Either way, you should be proactively looking to avoid an argument with your partner by finding the solution to the problems you are experiencing.

Never make the mistake of threatening your relationship or marriage when you argue because this is a guarantee of a break-up. When you have an argument and threatened to end things with your partner, you effectively place them in flight mode, and they feel too uncomfortable being around you.

A partner can easily make other plans, such as moving to another place if their relationship has been threatened. You might not mean to break up with them but using an argument to threaten the relationship should be motivation enough for you to avoid it because it guarantees the end of the relationship.

Research suggests that couples who spend more than twenty percent of their time together arguing will eventually break up. You have to understand the devastating consequences of arguments in relationships because they inevitably lead to both of you breaking up.

It should provide enough motivation for you to resolve problems in the most reasonable manner possible.

Chapter 3- Non-Violent Communication

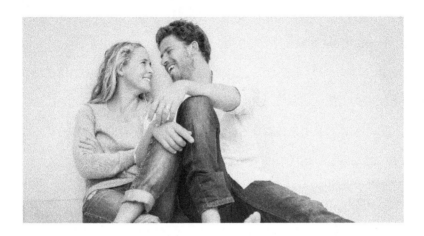

Stuff is bound to flare up in your relationships. There will be times when things will become so thick that people cannot see eye to eye, and this is when nonviolent communication (NVC) will come into play.

NVC prevents conflicts from taking place by establishing a foundation of respect and trust when people communicate. The great of NVC is that even at the point when you feel most angry and ready to flare up, NVC causes you to act in a trusting and respectful manner, without a hint of passive aggression that typically causes resentment and distrust.

By definition, NVC is a communication framework designed to reduce conflict and tension among people. It provides us with a lens that gives us an entirely different perspective of the world. It also changes how people express themselves to others, connect and communicate with others, and how they empathize with them. Essentially, NVC enables you to create a better, higher quality connection so that people may enjoy being in a relationship that has mutually beneficial outcomes.   Below are a few of the features of an NVC:

Peaceful Resolution of Conflicts

Conflicts are a normal part of interacting and relating with other people. Still, the important thing is to resolve them peacefully and productively, and this process requires some considerable time, support, and lots of practice. Peaceful conflict resolution engages both parties and has them working together to de-escalate, process, and resolve a conflict situation.

Instead of confronting each other or burying the conflict as a whole, feuding persons are encouraged to demonstrate courage by opening up to each other regarding the conflict and how it affected them. They are also asked to show compassion to each other's side of the story, empathizing with the other party's experiences or interpretation of the events. Thirdly, the parties are asked to work together, in collaboration, to process the conflict and to come up with a resolution plan. Here are the guidelines that help to chatter the way as you work towards resolving your conflict in a peaceful, healthy, and kind way, even in very tense circumstances:

Remain Calm

Remember that you control your emotions and not the other way. You must be able to manage your anger emotions before you can help another person manage his. Whichever method you use, from breathing deeply to others you may have up your sleeve, the idea here is to keep your emotions under wraps long enough to allow negotiation.

There Are No Winners

Sometimes, the conflict will revolve around a ridiculous issue of little or no consequence. For example, do not get caught up in conflict regarding a football match that happened or is going to happen. Although fans can be very passionate, the players determine which team wins and which ones lose by playing in the field. As fans, you have to sit back and watch. Do not lose your peace over things you have no control over, especially those that do not require your participation. Also, do not fear to submit to another's opinions regarding issues because they do not influence your life in the first place.

Give the Audience to The Other Party

If someone makes you part of an uncomfortable conversation, allow them to speak as much as they need to. Acting disinterested or interrupting them while they will not work in your favor only aggravates the situation. Remember that the person is not rational at the time, and he can pull you in that direction. Therefore, give him time to get everything off his system, and eventually, things will calm down.

Do Not Engage in Verbal Insults

when resolving a conflict, be watchful of your tone and the words you use. Avoid abusive or angry words; let your inner voice do the work. Audibly speaking profanity, screaming, and using hateful language only escalates the conflict.

Maintain A Safe and Comfortable Distance

If you fear that the situation could quickly deteriorate and turn physical, keep a safe distance from the other person. It will keep the person from attacking you or from interpreting your physical moves as offensive postures. Therefore, keep your distance and do not give room for the other person to feel threatened.

Overall, when you want to resolve a conflict peacefully, seek higher ground. Ask yourself, "Is it better to be right or happy?" From there, you will quickly figure out what you need to do.

Reconciliation After A Conflict

After a conflict, reconciliation allows parties to return to working together to build the society and achieve shared goals. Parties must begin to move past their divided opinions into a shared future. Reconciliation is meant to restore the relationship between people to allow for future engagements and collaborations. Unfortunately, reconciliation can be quite difficult, especially because there are so many setbacks and failures involved, depending on the conflict's depth. However, the only real failure would be if the parties involved did not consider reconciliation.

There is no definite systematic process that parties can follow to resolve a conflict; each situation demands a unique approach. However, there are some lessons you could carry away to help you resolve the conflicts in your life:

- Reconciliation is both the process and the destination.
- Reconciliation cannot be done in haste because it takes time to address the underlying issues such as anger, pain, frustration, etc.
- Reconciliation processes should not be judged as either successes or failures because each process will have its micro wins and successes.
- Reconciliation is done in several stages, and parties should expect relapses too.
- Mutual interests can be very effective in facilitating reconciliation between feuding parties.

With the understanding that reconciliation does not involve specific steps, parties should, however, ensure that both sides are heard. Parties must also be ready to abandon their old beliefs.

Secrets of Mediating Knowledge

There will be situations where the only thing feuding parties can agree on is that they need a mediator's help. The mediator ought to be a neutral party, whose role is not to judge and declare the winner and the loser. His goal is to help the parties come to an understanding.

Mediation takes place in two stages. The first stage is the joint session. Mediation begins by holding a meeting that lets the mediator in the prevailing situation. The parties present their facts, and each side indicates what its ideal resolution of the situation would be. The mediator also needs to have all the information regarding what started the conflict and where it has gotten.

The second stage is the caucus stage, and in this one, the mediator is obliged to hold separate sessions with each party. The meeting's details should be highly confidential, but for the statements that the first party would want to be repeated to the second party. The mediator then collects each side's interests, including information about the concerns and needs that the dispute is affecting.

Once the second stage is done, the mediator begins moving from one party to another, collecting proposals and suggestions that the parties believe will satisfy their interests equally. Ultimately, a solution is reached. Sometimes, it will be a one-sided victory, while other times, it will end in a 'win-win' situation.

Making Bad Thoughts Disappear

When bad thoughts plague your mind, close your eyes as tightly as you can, do not shut them out. The thought or the feeling keeps popping up, over and over. The thoughts could be of a disturbing story you heard on the news, nagging self-doubt, or thoughts of your relationship that went sour. All these thoughts make you miserable and cause you to feel imprisoned by your cruel mind.

Some people believe in the divine and will invoke their deities' power to drive the negative thoughts away, while the second group believes that nothing can be done about it. They believe that these thoughts have to come up and that blocking them out is only a waste of time. Now you can block out unproductive thoughts, but only when armed with the right strategies.

You must remember that blocking out the negative thoughts is an effort in futility because the thoughts rebound one way or another. When your guard is down, the thought comes back with the vengeance of a battalion, and suddenly, all you can think about are the negative thoughts. However, it is possible to block out the negative thoughts and not have any rebounds; you only need to remember two things.

The first is that blocking the thought is difficult, but just because it is difficult does not mean that you need to think about it. Your brain is not out to get you with the negativities. Stop thinking about the difficulty of letting the thoughts go because it is this thinking that gives the thought more meaning and importance, making it even more challenging to get rid of.

The second step is to know how to handle negative thought when it shows up. The solution is to plan, in advance, what to do when the thought comes to mind. Some opt to ignore it, while others choose to replace the negative thought with some positive ones.

Using Positive Language

Language is quite a powerful tool, and how you express yourself affects how it is received, whether positively or negatively. Positive language is so effective it is used to convey even bad news. It also elicits cooperation and reception, unlike negative language that arouses confrontation and argument. In your daily communication, positive language helps project a positive, helpful image, while negative language projects a destructive image.

You must have come across a naysayer in the course of your life. A naysayer is a person who criticizes ideas, always having an opinion about why an idea will not work. Sometimes, the naysayer will not even have a negative attitude; they will speak using words or a tone that implies negativity. If you have been around someone like that, you know just how annoying and mentally fatiguing a person like that can be.

Since naysayers get creative by the day, here is how you identify negative language: it carries the message that you cannot do something, it subtly blames you, it does not mention or stress the positive consequences, and it includes words like cannot, unable to, won't, and other words that let the listener or the reader know what cannot be done.

On the other hand, the positive language will tell you what can be done; it will sound encouraging or helpful than bureaucratic, offer suggestions of possible alternatives, and stresses the positive actions or consequences that the reader or listener should expect. You certainly would want to lean towards positive language so that you can be a fountain of hope and positivity for others. Take up positive language and positive thinking and replace all your negative statements with positive ones.

Chapter 4- Loving Words Heal Relationships

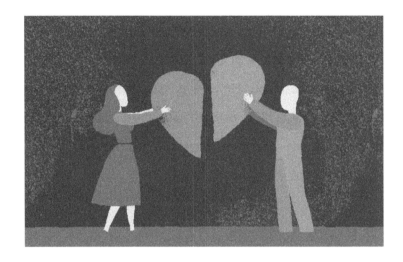

The most dominant two phrases that heal a harmed relationship are the two phrases that are hardest to state, "I'm Sorry" and "I was wrong." It is basic in healing relationships for couples.

The motivation behind why these phrases are hardest to state is because we would prefer not to admit that we have caused whatever broke or harmed a relationship. More often than not, we say that it was the other person's deficiency. Also, we hang tight for that person to be the first to apologize. In any case, the apology never comes because the other person is likewise hanging tight for it.

What's more, we realize that relationships inside the family and outside of it sometimes end in the absence of this apology. We know many separations happen just because either never made a move to apologize.

For what reason is it so challenging to admit that we weren't right and to apologize? It is straightforward that it is a human instinct, a shortcoming that puts us over the others. What we need is to defeat this commitment to self. It requires personal development, compassion, and thinking about the other. What's more, a necessary apology will reestablish that broken relationship.

It doesn't make a difference who fouled up when a relationship is broken. Significantly, we venture out. Remember that the other person feels a similar way. We should state something that can prompt healing, for example, "I'm sorry that we are having this issue. Would we be able to discuss making things right once more?"

Making a stride like this quite often prompts healing a broken relationship. Furthermore, more often than not, the conversation results in the two gatherings saying 'sorry,' which typically leads to a more grounded relationship.

Any healing in a relationship for couples requires some forgiveness. It should originate from the heart before it is said in words.

One must be cautious about like that as it may, in communicating forgiveness. To state "I forgive you" amidst a battle may be misjudged as "You weren't right," and would compound the situation. We should say "I forgive you" just when the other person requests forgiveness. At that point, these become the ideal words. Mercy can heal the relationship as well as the bodies and the brains of the two persons. Keep in mind, in healing relationships for couples, we as of now have the words. We need to state them. Have an incredible relationship by utilizing words that heal.

Falling in Love - Through Your Own Love Words

Whether you have begun to look all starry-eyed years prior or hoping to become hopelessly enamored now, we can share some extremely sentimental approaches to share your emotions. Purchasing a love card or a romantic ballad is excellent; in any case, words mean more when you get them directly from your own heart. You need to realize how to state what you might want to express. From that point forward, applying some inventiveness will make you incline that your beginning to look all starry-eyed just because.

- Address it with the right "pet name."
- Use detail, and don't be hesitant to get "mushy."
- Express yourself enthusiastically with love quotes
- Be inventive and unique include something new.

When writing to the love of your life, it is great to start it off with a pet name. Perhaps you have something that nobody else hears? It would be the ideal time to use it. This love letter will be among you and the one you love, so make it individual. A few people like to use (infant, sweetie, hun, and so on).

When writing a sentimental love letter, it is tied in with being mushy. Express yourself now with all the soft stuff that you typically don't state. Try not to keep down, after this is the thing that a love letter is about. Get energetic with your words, and let that individual recognize what your heart feels for them.

Presently, someplace in the middle of the letter, use their real name. You would prefer not to overdo it by a considerable amount of pet names, yet one to start, and real name in the middle ought to be great. Make sure to use love quotes all through this gem. Genuine romance does not come around over and over again. You need to make sure you treat it well and care for it while you have it. You're telling them you love them, with imaginative detail.

Include something new. Something you have not raised in quite a while, or at no other time. Demonstrate to them that something new emerges to you. State what your heart needed to shout, the day you realized you were in love. Connections can be precarious, yet if you enable yourself to recollect how much you are in love, you will do fine.

How to Express Love Words

Communicating to a person that you genuinely like calls for the use of love words. Love is the single component that makes a society what it is. Without love, there is no life, which is why words of love are significant. There are numerous things that best display love words, and when the name is referenced, many recognize what it implies. People use multiple ways and incorporate the words and; they can do it orally, or they can write it down. The vast majority, when they were growing up, used to write love letters to one another. Today, people keep on composing love letters. It is an instrument used to display love words. It is a rare occurrence natural to impart these words, and it calls for certified fondness. There is something men do that best express the words. Initially, understand that words are simply words if there is no activity to coordinate. It is likely the best thing about love. Love is best shown in any case when words are included. It affirms what there, as of now, is.

In this manner, if you wish to use the words, you must reexamine yourself and see if you love the person. Sentimental love between a man and a lady is what we have portrayed above, and a portion of the words you will discover incorporate the accompanying. Dear sweetheart, nectar, my love, my favorite, and the list go on. Love is dynamic, and people are inventive. New ages keep on concocting love words like baby, boo, and numerous others. When it comes to utilizing these words, you must ensure that the person you are communicating with gets it. When there is viable correspondence, you can likewise anticipate just useful things in your relationship. There are such vast numbers of love words that you can use, and different societies and even religions may decide the words. Different dialects will have their one-of-a-kind arrangement of words. While you wish to express your love to somebody, it doesn't need to be sexual love. You can have respect for your children, guardians, sisters, etc. It is additionally extremely vital to express appreciation to such people, and many do it consistently.

Next to a portion of the words that people use to demonstrate their children love pumpkin, bear, love bear, daylight, baby, and the list goes on. You can think of your one-of-a-kind words, which can be a nickname and is equipped with love. It is important to be active in showing love to other people. In society, some people frequently feel dismissed. Such people might not have dear companions or family. Life is desolate when you have nobody to impart to, and you ought to endeavor to make love any place and whenever conceivable. If you're the sort of person who isn't active in showing love, begin doing as such, and you don't need to write a love letter. It is the thing that you state and how you state it. Love can include numerous viewpoints and figure out how to radiate through your cooperative attitude.

Using Words of Love to Inspire the Relationship - 3 Tips for Men to Learn

Relationships are a back and forth movement in the life of many of us as we clear our path through the riddles of life and of love. To live in the steady fight is to live in the bogus acknowledgment that by one way or another, there are always victors and failures as we cross the minefield of love.

We come at it from an altogether different point of view as we take a gander at the words we as a whole appear to use to get us to where we even have a relationship. Men, generally, need such a considerable amount of assistance in this field and typically wallow because of poor role models, societal impacts, peer pressure, and only by and large sluggishness in needing to be something more with their words their partner.

There is always a way out, yet numerous men neglect to search for the way in any case when talking love to their partner. So, what are a few ways to make words mean things again with your partner? A couple of tips can always prove to be useful, right men?

Tip 1:

Women need to hear your heart. It is most likely one of the hardest things for men to do due to the reality they were never educated. Begin little here, folks — an all-around set note left before work can be an incredible beginning. The significant thing to do here is to claim your powerlessness to share your heart NOW yet disclose to her that you are learning.

Tip 2:

Not each cherishing word should lead to sex! What a stunning man. Because you state something decent doesn't imply that the spoken words are S-E-X! Get over yourself. In some cases, the most sentimental things we do will never lead to sex, nor should they.

Tip 3:

Love to love. Reevaluate your relationship as a way to love simply cherishing your partner. If you center around your identity's quintessence as a team, the relationship will rule your faculties.

Keep in mind, men. You are more than what you at any point, though you were with your words. Presently, live that way. At last, love is all there is, so let your words be your beginning.

Chapter 5- The Role and Importance of Empathy in Your Relationship

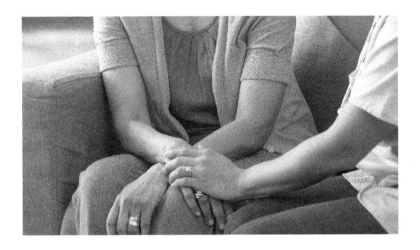

People tend to confuse empathy with sympathy. However, you need to know the difference between the two. To have compassion for someone means to feel pity or sorrow for them when they face some misfortune. To have empathy means being able to understand and share their feelings.

It is typical for people to disagree with each other on things. Everyone has their own opinions and feelings. However, it is important to respect the other person's feelings and not try to railroad over them with your own. It is especially so in a relationship. You have to cultivate a sense of compassion and endure the other person's views and emotions. Empathy will allow you to do this and develop a strong relationship with your partner.

Influence of Empathy in A Relationship

You need to have empathy for your partner, and they should do the same for you too. When you can empathize with another person, you will feel what they are feeling in some way. For instance, you will understand their pain or feel happy when they are happy. If you can develop empathy within yourself, you will perceive your partner's emotions even as they keep changing. It is crucial to help you understand each other and provide support when they need it. Having empathy will help you become more compassionate. Developing compassion in yourself is important as it will make you want to help your partner in their time of need and provide them with the care they require. If you fail to have empathy for the other person, you will not have compassion for them either. It is because you will fail to recognize their emotions and thus fail to react appropriately too. According to many studies, people who lack empathy are usually the ones who are mean to others. They fail to understand how their words and actions affect the other person. Such people lie to themselves and refuse to take responsibility for their actions. They rarely show remorse for hurting another person. It can harm all their relationships in life regardless of whether it is at work or home.

Empathy is actually at the heart of a happy relationship. Your relationship will struggle to survive when it lacks empathy. You will lack compassion without empathy, and this will affect the bond you have with your partner. Empathy is like a bridge between two individuals who have different feelings, thoughts, or perspectives. Empathy can be of three types.

Cognitive empathy is when you can look at things from another person's perspective but cannot feel their emotions. It will allow you to appreciate a situation the other person is going through.

Emotional empathy allows you to feel what the other person is feeling or thinking. It allows you to connect with the person more emotionally.

Compassionate empathy is a balance of both cognitive plus emotional empathy. It allows you to see things from the other person's perspective and empathize with their emotions.

Compassionate empathy is what you need to develop to a greater extent within yourself. Cognitive or emotional empathy can often have a negative impact. For instance, someone can use it to manipulate someone for their benefit. But with compassionate empathy, you will feel compassion and be less inclined to want to harm anyone. If you have compassionate empathy, you will think twice before you do anything and be more considerate of your partner's feelings. If you know that your partner feels annoyed or frustrated when the room is messy, you will empathize and keep it clean. Your empathy will help you become a good partner, and they will appreciate your efforts. Compassionate empathy will help you respond to your partner with love, compassion, and understanding.

How to Develop Empathy

Now that you recognize the importance of it, you should try to nurture empathy within yourself. The following steps will help you in becoming more empathetic.

Increase your self-awareness. When you become more attuned to your own emotions and thoughts, you will also recognize these in others. If something hurts you, you will know that it could hurt another person too. Take notice of how you feel and think when your partner is saying or doing something. Don't be too absorbed in yourself and learn to exert control over the way you react.

Practice self-empathy. You will fail to empathize with your partner when you cannot sympathize with yourself. You need to pay attention to your own emotions and acknowledge when you are going through a difficult time. Taking care of yourself should always be a priority. Don't compromise self-care in an attempt to take care of your partner. You can face your issues without catastrophic about it. Remaining calm and composed will help you meet everything that comes your way.

Pay attention to body language. Be careful about your body language and learn to observe that of others as well. A person's gestures, expressions, and various movements can tell a lot about their feelings.

Observe nonverbal cues. How a person says, something is often more revealing than what they are saying. The nonverbal cues will help to identify their emotional truth.

Develop the habit of listening well. You won't empathize with someone if you don't even listen to what they are saying. Pay attention to the details, and be a good listener. Avoid interrupting someone when they talk. Give them an opportunity to express themselves freely. Too many people are focused on talking more than listening. Give genuine attention to your partner at all times. Even when you argue, don't be focused on finding a way to defend yourself. Focus on what they are saying and try to understand their perspective.

Look for the positive aspects of your partner and your relationship. When you concentrate too much on the negative, you affect your ability to empathize healthily. Start taking note of the good things instead of constantly thinking of the bad.

Avoid being judgmental or doubting what the other person says. Listen with an open heart and mind. Don't focus too much on giving advice or telling them what they should or should not do. When a person shared their problem, they trust you and are looking for support. You should be more focused on listening than trying to solve the problem. Keep your own opinions and values aside and focus on what the other person feels and needs from you. Being too entangled in your perspective will prevent you from acting mindfully toward your partner.

Use these tips to develop a sense of empathy for your partner and others. It will make a lot of difference in how you communicate with people, and it will positively improve your relationships with them.

How to Communicate with Empathy

Now that you understand a little more about empathy, you have to start communicating with it in mind. If you are experiencing finding the right things to say, the following statements might help you figure it out.

Acknowledge your partner's pain. You need to acknowledge how they feel at all times. They will feel supported when you connect with their struggle or pain. You may use the following sentences:

- "I am sorry that you have to go through this."
- "I hate that this happened to you."
- "This must be hard for you."

- "I can see that this must be a difficult situation for you."

Share your feelings. You can be truthful and admit it when you don't know what to say or do. It is not always easy to imagine what the other person is going through. Share your thoughts and let your partner know that you are trying. You may use the following sentences:

- "I wish I could make things better."
- "My heart hurts for you."
- "I'm really sad that this happened to you."
- "I'm sorry that you are feeling this way."

Show your partner that you are grateful when they open up to you. People find it difficult to open up and be vulnerable to others. More often than not, their trust has been broken at some point. So when they choose to trust you, you need to be grateful and express it. Show your partner you appreciate that they share their thoughts and emotions with you. Acknowledge how difficult it can be for them to do this sometimes. You may use the following sentences:

- "I'm glad that you shared this with me."
- "I'm glad that you are telling me this."

- "I can imagine how hard it must be to talk about this. Thank you for sharing it with me."
- "I appreciate you trying to work hard on our relationship. I know you are trying, and that gives me hope."

Show your partner that you are interested in. You have to take an interest in what your partner is going through. It can be hard to go through difficult times alone. You have to reach out and show them that you are there for support. Show them that you are listening to whatever they have to say. Don't offer too much advice or too many opinions. Just be a good listener. You may use the following sentences:

- "How are you feeling about all that's been going on lately?"
- "I think you're feeling like ——. Am I right? Did I misunderstand?"
- "What has this been like for you?"

Show encouragement. When your partner or spouse is going through a tough time, you have to be encouraging. But you need to go about this the right way. Don't try to fix their problem or offer unsolicited advice. Just encourage them in a way that makes them feel better and motivated. Show them that you care and that you believe in them. You may use the following sentences:

- "You are strong, and I believe you can get through this."
- "I am always on your side. You should never feel alone."
- "I'm proud of everything that you have done."
- "You matter, and you should never question it."
- "You are a very talented person."

Chapter 6- Showing Gratitude

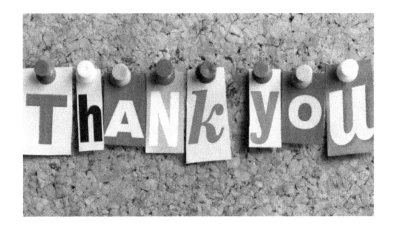

Expressing appreciation is perhaps the best way to reassure your companion that you value them, with some great bonuses. Partners who are soulmates have also discovered forms of communicating appreciation that go beyond a mere "thank you."

If both you and your companion search for different forms to incorporate this wonderful practice into your romantic life, look no farther than this part.

Gratitude is essential since it strengthens connections. Evidence not only indicates that showing appreciation helps us feel better overall (which may have a significant effect on the relationship itself), but it has often been shown to contribute to longer and more loving relationships.

It only makes sense in the best relationships to be appreciative of your mate and to show it.

Frequent appreciation shows your companion that you value them and act as a reminder of the special position in your life. Everybody needs to be acknowledged, and hence the relationship will be improved overall. Beyond these two simple words, there are several ways to convey the emotion behind "thank you", and professionals know just what they are.

How to Express Gratitude

Send Text Messages for No Reason

Texting does not seem like an important part of a relationship, but looking at how partners text each other can tell you a lot about their relationship (how they treat one another and what they feel about each other).

Sending a text without any reason can be a big sign of gratitude. If anyone, including our partners, thinks of us out of the blue, it shows us that we have value in their eyes and that the choices we do make have enduring beneficial results. And if you're searching for new methods to show your companion how much they mean to you, give them a "thinking about you" randomly. It could make their day.

Constantly Acknowledge the Smallest of Things

Gratitude is always expressed in its purest nature when a partner understands the day-to-day effort that their companion invests into their life or relationship.

Gratitude involves acknowledging the small things that mostly stop getting noticed. Not only getting the garbage out or changing the bed also, anytime you see your companion try when they're exhausted, or acknowledging the role they have in your family or life.

Acknowledging something about our companion that they thought you didn't even notice generates a strong bond. Often people in life ignore the tasks that their companions perform in having things function smoothly. Very happy partners seemed to have no such problem.

Perform Active Listening

Couples that are thankful to each other seem to be more involved in the moment with each other.

Gratitude can involve being engaged in discussions by active listening, listening through all our senses, rather than only awaiting our turn to talk.

If we are genuinely heard, we feel appreciated. Effectively listening to others is a beautiful expression of appreciation and love. It can also manifest in conflicts, with the pair not talking to each other, with each person genuinely wanting to grasp the other's view. It is not easy, of course, but it is a way to prove that you appreciate your partner even when you are angry.

Publicly Praise Them

It could be sharing a Facebook or Instagram post about your partner's work achievements (# humblebrag), or informing your mom how good the food your partner makes is, or how they aced their presentation last week while you're all together. Not only will this make your companion know how truly proud you are for them and their success, but it will also help you realize how fortunate you are to be alongside them.

Seek Ways to Offer Authentic Compliments

If you're in a long-term partnership, you probably understand clearly what you and your companion like about the other; sharing these feelings is an essential part of showing your appreciation.

Choose something you admire about the other and praise your partner. Individuals who feel valued by their partners feel happier, appreciated, and attractive. Conveying this type of affection means informing your companion when you think of them positively and seeking opportunities for them to realize that it comes from a really deep position of love.

Generate Openness

Experts believe that there's a general sense of warmth between the involved individuals in a grateful relationship. Strong partners often demonstrate that they respect each other as their interactions, body language, and mannerisms are usually warm and welcoming. Their faces brighten as they do small stuff for each other, and they respond enthusiastically, which demonstrates appreciation even though it's undisclosed. Thus, gratitude is not only in the stuff that you do but also in how you portray yourself.

If you're not sure how to get going with this, a light smile may do the trick. Only showing your wife a soft and heartfelt smile, as a way to show appreciation, will make a lot of difference. They would certainly know what you think.

Make Sacrifices

Another means of showing appreciation is making sacrifices for your beloved, no matter how simple they may be. Sacrifice is a perfect way to express gratitude, and thus, good couples constantly make sacrifices. Your companion may, for example, work 40 + hours a week to cover the bills, so you abandon your usual Saturday plans to spend time with them since it is their day off. You don't have to sacrifice your lifestyle very much for them, but you should make small changes now and then prove you care.

Write to Them

The love letters needn't be a relic of the past. And even if you think you're not eloquent, a little note will go a long way in your relationship. A handwritten letter or a cute card can help in expressing that you value your partner. Just think how valued you'd feel if your partner gives you a love letter.

It's also very special to hang onto a letter or a sheet of paper with the handwriting on it, and it demonstrates to your partner you've taken the time out of the day to focus on something special for them. It is particularly poignant if their language of love is receiving presents.

Directly Say It

Just telling your companion exactly what you are grateful for regarding them also works. There's no need to beat around or be careful with your words. Often, it's best to be direct. Solid couples are direct about their appreciation stating things like "I'm very thankful to you for assisting me with my chores" or something equally unambiguous.

Be specific in your thanks. If you praise your companion, be descriptive about it. Exactly inform them why you admire their contributions and how it strengthens your life and happiness. You can express your affection to your companion in many respects, but this one will be effective, even though it seems simple.

Express Gratitude Creatively

"Thank you" is a successful starting but not always strong enough. If you agree that "all is fine in moderation", then you recognize that hearing "thank you" can so much lack its well-intentioned importance.

Even changing the word selection affects how valued the mate feels. You can create a difference by saying, "I love it when you..." or "It makes me so happy that you..." Even besides using terms, talk of the forms you might express your thanks instead of saying them.

Preparing their favorite meal during a busy work week or having them go to bed early while you take care of the children are little ways to reassure your companion that you are thankful for their tireless efforts. Bringing home roses or their preferred chocolate on a special day can always make them feel loved, and putting a note on the refrigerator is also a fun way to say thank you, which means more than just verbal thanks.

Expressions of appreciation are essential to a healthy relationship, irrespective of how they want to express it. Soulmates show these emotions to each other in several forms, from kisses to love notes, but they all say one thing: Thank you.

Chapter 7- Revisit Family

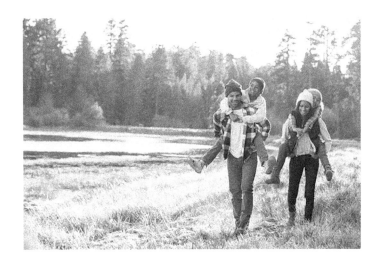

Parenting is a game-changer to all marriages. In many ways, it can change the relationship dynamic for the better or worse, depending on the specific set of circumstances. In television commercials featuring baby-shower cards, diapers, and a litany of baby products, parenting and marriage are depicted as pure bliss and effortless. Your relatives will sell you a story about how babies are a heaven-sent bundle of happiness – and they are – but they skip the hard work that goes into making it all work!

Of course, it is essential to love our children. But it is crucial to be alive to what parenting does to marriages. There is no reason that loving your child and working on your marriage should be mutually exclusive. A happy marriage almost always means a happy baby. Marriage happiness, sustainability, and worth are liked at the hip with parenting.

Studies into the relationship between marriage and parenting indicate that most relationships change for the worse when couples transition into families. Initially, caring for the baby means sleepless nights, a surge in demands in bringing up the baby, and an abundance of new expectations for both parents. The parents also have to hold down the requirements of a job. Between 30 and 50 percent of couples that become parents face massive stress and depression.

University of California, Berkeley researchers, establish that more than 70 percent of all new mothers faced a marked decline in marital satisfaction. Around one-third of new mothers and fathers experience substantial depression after becoming parenting. One-eighth of all couples who transition into parents experience divorce when their babies hit 18 months.

Shifting from lovers to parents can be tumultuous to your marriage. The transition shakes the foundations of your relations. The result is a massive disruption of the normal flow of information between partners. It also upends the status quo of emotions and individual responsibilities. In short, there is a learning curve for the lovers when they become parents. Completing the learning and adjusting accordingly is vital to the success of parenting and marriage.

The emotional disruption is mainly driven by the changes in the typical social dynamics. For example, a working mom's life shifts from the bubbly office colleagues for breastfeeding, dealing with laundry mountains, and bottle-washing.

After around six months, she faces the prospect of changing back to her working routine. The husband has to work with the wife through the entire process. However, most fathers feel left out of the early years of caring for the child. The overall result is each of the spouses is doing more, the communication lines and frequency declines, and both feel massively underappreciated.

As the kid grows, you suddenly wonder if your child will be enrolled in the right preschool program. You worry whether your daughter or son is in the right music, art, and tumbling tots' classes.

Can Parenting Be Used to Strength Marriages?

It is not easy. It isn't easy. But marriage can be used to sweeten your marriage, make it stronger and long-lasting! Most people view parenting as a collection of stressors that will make your life miserable and probably accelerate the end of your relationship with your spouse. However, with the right touch, parenting can be the glue that holds you together. In this regard, it will benefit your relationship and the well-being of the kid(s).

All you can do to leverage parenting in improving your relationship within a marriage is to put your relationship first. Recognizing that your marriage is a work in progress goes a long way to cementing your commitment towards bolstering your bonds. Working on your differences consistently also helps strengthen your relationship's foundations while ironing out disagreements before they become more significant issues.

A focus on appreciating each other while minimizing criticism is essential in sweetening your relationship. Communication is the underlying foundation of a relationship. Maintaining the bidirectional flow of information, opinions, views, and perspectives is necessary, retaining the enthusiasm to sustain a relationship of married spouses with a kid(s).

Using parenting as a tool to improve your relationship quality and sustainability needs a deliberate effort targeting parenting dynamics. Understanding the expected disruptions to the relationship parenting brings will help you be better prepared. It also means that you are better equipped to harness the parenting changes and work for your relationship.

Learning about parenting and preparing for the shifts it brings should include both spouses. This process must be collaborative because both of you will need the knowledge and skills to maneuver through the impending changes. Secondly, a concerted approach is likely to succeed in maintaining a working and effective relationship. When both of you put in the work, you are susceptible to shoulder the burden equitably. Although parenting cannot biologically be equitable, it creates a sense that the husband is supportive of the wife during this period.

The challenge facing most couples going into marriage is that they are not prepared for parenting disruptions. They are not ready to spend their lives after the baby is born and parenting begins. As a result, parenting becomes overwhelming, physically, and emotionally. It leads to a surge in conflicts and an increase in the likelihood of divorce or unhappy marriages/relationships. Here are some ways on how you can use parenting as a platform to build a stronger and long-lasting relationship and marriage:

Talk About the Certainties and Uncertainties Ahead

Talking about uncertainties does not make them any more confident. However, it will help you be emotionally prepared and sure of yourself when navigating through parenting moments and circumstances.

It is also important to plan and ventilate some particular issues, such as splitting errands and household chores. It is essential to talk about where the income of the family will come from. In this case, it is crucial to answering the following questions: Who will be the breadwinner? And who is going to stay at home rearing the child?

Talk about the day-care option. Establish who will get your baby to the day-care center and who will get him/her back. Explore the issue of a babysitter, the budget for this option, and plan your lives around what you agree. Figure out how night shift duties will be split, who will wash or sterilize the breast pump and bottles daily. Figure out the shopping schedule, cooking plan, and cleaning chores.

These details seem small and harmless. But without figuring out the division of labor regarding these aspects, they might contribute to frustration, stress, and depression. If left unsorted, they can gnaw away at the relationship.

However, figuring them out creates an understanding and collaborative approach that is healthy for your relationship. It also establishes a sense that everyone is doing their fair share. Moreover, developing a concise plan for dealing with these chores and duties reduces the chances that you will be overwhelmed as a couple when parenting begins. Emotionally, you will be prepared for the deluge of tasks and responsibilities, which will make it markedly more comfortable to handle and transition into the parenting role.

Focus on the Downside of Parenthood with the View of Avoiding its Pitfalls on the Marriage

Maintaining a positive and hopeful perception of parenting is important for new fathers and mothers. But it is vital to guard against lofty expectations shattered by the reality of fatherhood and motherhood.

Yes, babies offer massive joy, and they bring a lot of happiness to a marriage. They also carry an uptick in physical and emotional exertions that can take their toll on the relationship. Bathing the baby, feeding, entertaining, and changing the baby 24 hours a day and 7 hours a week are demanding chores. All couples should be emotionally and physically prepared for such demands before they begin their roles as parents.

Focusing on and talking about the downside(s) of parenting is essential in marriage. It will help you to cope with the changes and disruptions to your lives. It is okay to talk about your fatigue, frustrations, and even anger with your spouse. Ensure, to be honest with your partner regarding these issues and also maintaining a supportive stance.

Feeling anger, frustration, and fatigue does not mean that you are a terrible parent. It is crucial to admit these emotions and focus on working together to resolve them within the marriage. This approach helps in disarming these emotions and thus prevents them from negatively affecting your relationship.

For example, you can agree in advance that if one of you is overwhelmed and is unable to fulfill their chores, the other will cover and take care of the baby for a while. It provides an option of relief for the overwhelmed partner. It also establishes a mutually supportive dynamic that deepens your affection for each other amid a challenging period.

Fatigue, frustrations, and even anger resulting from anger can marinate into more significant marriage issues. For example, these emotions can easily lead to resentment of each other, lack of trust, and a communication breakdown. By focusing on constant and honest communication, you will always know how your partner is feeling at all times. You can render your support when they need it and shoulder some of their fear and uncertainty.

Maintain Honesty About Gains and Losses

In many instances, parenting will lead to some gains and losses. For example, you have gained the baby of your dreams. He/she melts your heart every time you see them. However, you cannot avoid feeling sad and empty because of the loss of your typical sex life. For the mother, you lost your sleek pre-baby size 8s and replaced them with elastic-waist jeans.

Most new parents typically complain, silently, about the disruption to their lives occasioned by the baby and their parenting duties and responsibilities. These complaints and silent resentment cause the marital distance to widen. In some extreme instances, it can lead to shame and a decline in self-esteem.

For example, a new daddy might feel replaced by the baby in his spouse's life and affection. The mother might be frustrated and even sad about how parenting (pregnancy, nursing, and the rigors of childcare) has transformed her body. These feelings are normal among new parents.

Sharing such feelings of loss, shame, or disruption is vital in dealing with parenting's emotional toll. Maintaining honesty about these issues with your partner helps you to feel better and strengthen your bond as a couple.

Communication regarding these feelings helps establish a perspective for behavior. For example, feelings of loss might make the mother snappy and frustrated, which might spill over to her interactions with other people, including the husband. The husband might also display emotions and reactions that are out of the norm.

Through communication and honesty, you will sort through these emotions and explain the context of behavior. The resulting understanding will create rigor room for a learning curve and some space for your relationship's growth and development.

Chapter 8- Spice Up Your Sex Life

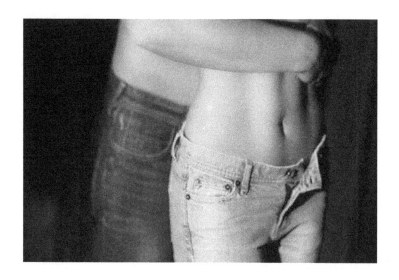

We spent many times in this guide learning about communication and how it can help improve your relationship. Now it's time to take it to a new level and improve aspects of your sex life. It is especially important for those who have been in a relationship with the same person for some time. Things may start to feel a bit dull, and sex drives may not be as strong as they used to be. It is the perfect time to start rebuilding that sexual relationship with your partner by trying new things, communicating about personal desires, and playing fun games. In this part, we will be exploring the following topics; increasing couple intimacy, spicing up your sex life, trying new positions, playing new games, and communicating your sexual wants/needs.

Increase Couple Intimacy

As your relationship progresses, it is essential to keep sex and lust alive. When you become progressively more comfortable with someone, it can take away some of the mystery. It is because there is no longer the excitement of getting to know a person and having everything you do together be brand new. At the beginning of a relationship, you are eager to have sex with each other because the other person is new and hot and a novelty of sorts. As you get used to them, it can be easy to lose those feelings and settle into the comfortability of everything (like their body or your routine). It is by no means a bad thing. Getting to this point in your relationship is fun and comforting in its way and is different from but better than the early stages. From a sexual perspective, though, we don't want the coming of this stage of your relationship to bring with it the end of exciting sex life.

If you are a long-term or married couple, you have likely tried every one of the classic sex positions together, from missionary to 69. You have probably also developed a routine of your favorite positions and the order in which you do them by now. While you probably know how to please each other like it's second nature, rediscovering each other's bodies in a sexy way and learning new ways to pleasure each other is good for couples who have been together for a long time.

In the beginning, you may have started having sex casually before you got together romantically, or you may have begun having sex when you became a couple. Either way, the beginning of any relationship comes with a lot of uncharted territories. You are exploring a new person's entire body- inside and out, and letting them see all of yours. Of course, this can be nerve-wracking. There will be some positions and sexual activities that you won't be completely comfortable doing with this person yet, even if you have done them before with someone else. There are certain positions you can stick to that are more comfortable at the beginning of a relationship, and that is best for getting to know someone's body and what they like. These positions serve us well when we are newly having sex with a person and are looking for the best way to help each other orgasm. You may think that you are well past this stage in a long-term relationship. This stage of discovery, however, is something that we want to return to every so often. We want to rediscover the person's body and what they like as if it is the first time we are exploring it. People's desires change, and their bodies change. It is important to continue to know how to pleasure your partner as they grow and change and to expect the same from them for yourself. Further, revisiting our partner's body with an open mind as if we know nothing about it can be a fun and flirty way to renew zest in your sex life.

Importance of Spicing Up Your Sex Life

The main importance of spicing up your sex life is to increase intimacy between you and your partner. Not only does this help your sex life become more fun and exciting, but it also improves the communication and bond between you and your partner. In this part, we will be examining intimacy and the role that it plays in romantic relationships. We will look at how you can work to maintain intimacy with your partner and what achieving a greater level of intimacy can and will do for your relationship.

Intimacy is very important between two people when part of a couple, especially in the bedroom. Intimacy is what brings you close and keeps you close. Firstly, we will look at what intimacy means and the different types of intimacy that exist. There are different types of intimacy, and here I will outline them for you before digging deeper into the intimacy between couples. Intimacy, in a general sense, is defined as mutual openness and vulnerability between two people. There are different ways in which you can give and receive openness and vulnerability in a relationship. Intimacy does not have to include a sexual relationship (though it can). Therefore, it is not only reserved for romantic relationships. Intimacy can also be present in other types of close relationships like friendships or family relationships. Below, we will outline the different forms of intimacy.

Emotional Intimacy

Emotional intimacy is the ability to express oneself maturely and openly, leading to a deep emotional connection between people. Saying things like "I love you" or "you are very important to me" are examples of this. It is also the ability to respond maturely and openly when someone expresses themselves to you by saying things like "I'm sorry" or "I love you too." This open and vulnerable dialogue leads to an emotional connection. There must be a mutual willingness to be vulnerable and open with one's deeper thoughts and feelings for a deep emotional connection to form. It is where this type of emotional intimacy comes from.

Intellectual Intimacy

Intellectual intimacy is a kind of intimacy that involves discussing and sharing thoughts and opinions on intellectual matters. They gain fulfillment and feelings of closeness with the other person. For example, if you discuss politics with someone you deem to be an intellectual equal, you may find that you feel a closeness with them as you share your thoughts and opinions and connect on an intellectual level. Many people find intellect and brains to be sexy in a partner!

Shared Interests and Activities

This form of intimacy is less well-known, but it is also considered a form of intimacy. When you share activities with another person, you both enjoy and are passionate about; this creates a sense of connection. For example, when you cook together or travel together. These shared experiences give you memories to share, leading to bonding and intimacy (openness and vulnerability). This type of connection is usually present in friendships, familial relationships, and, more importantly, in romantic relationships. Being able to share interests and activities leads to a closeness that can be defined as intimacy.

Physical Intimacy

Physical intimacy is the type that most people think of when they hear the term "intimacy," It is the kind that we will be most concerned with within this guide, as it is the type of intimacy that includes sex and all activities related to sex. It also involves other non-sexual types of physical contact, such as hugging and kissing. Physical intimacy can be found in close friendships or familial relationships where hugging and kisses on the cheek are common, but it is most often found in romantic relationships.

Physical intimacy is the type of intimacy involved when people are trying to make each other orgasm. Physical intimacy is almost always required for orgasm. Physical intimacy doesn't necessarily mean that you are in love with the person you are having sex with; it just means that you are doing something intimate with another person physically.

It is also possible to be intimate with yourself. While this begins with the emotional intimacy of self-awareness, it also involves the physical intimacy of masturbation and physical self-exploration. I define sexual, the physical intimacy of the self as being in touch with the parts of yourself physically that you would not normally be in touch with if you are a woman, your breasts, your clitoris, vagina, and your anus. Suppose you are a man, your testicles, your penis, your anus. Being physically intimate with yourself allows you to have more fulfilling sex, more fulfilling orgasms, and a more fulfilling overall relationship with your body. Allowing someone to be physically intimate with you in a sexual way is also an emotionally intimate experience, regardless of your relationship with the person. Being in charge of your own body while it is in the hands of another person is very important, and this is why masturbation is such a key element to physical intimacy.

You can think of physical intimacy as something that breaks the barrier of personal space. This definition includes touching of any sort, but especially sexual intercourse, kissing, touching, and anything else of a sexual nature. When you are having sex with anyone, regardless of whether you have romantic feelings for them or not, you are having a physically intimate relationship with them. The difference between a relationship that involves physical intimacy alone and a romantic relationship is that a romantic relationship will also involve emotional intimacy, shared activities, and intellectual intimacy. A deep and lasting romantic relationship will need to include all of these forms of intimacy at once.

Chapter 9- The Secrets to Meaningful Relationships

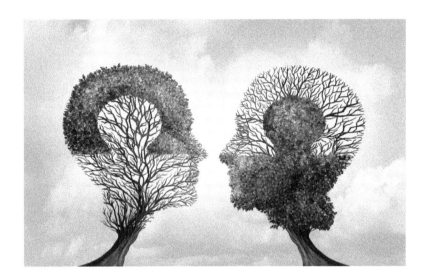

To have meaning in life alludes to whether one's actions are beneficial and are joined by a feeling of significant worth in one's achievements. Important relationships can assemble confidence and therefore fulfill us. They can likewise prompt fulfilling more significant level needs, for example, development and improvement.

There is a significant contrast between reason and importance. Knowing our motivation in life is imperative to satisfaction since it entirely grounds our behavior. Our motivation is the central persuading factor that gets us up during the first part of the day – i.e., our purpose behind being, which means it is worth allocating to that conviction. It has a worth direction, which means life has a moral segment to it. It rotates around how we treat others in our life.

Another significant differentiation is whether your relationships carry bliss and empower you to flourish. Important relationships advance our physical and psychological prosperity.

Glad life is one where we are happy with life's conditions, and it very well may be fortified by seriousness. A significant relationship is one that propels our prosperity, for instance, devoting ourselves to a beneficial goal. Together, they empower us to flourish.

One key to building important relationships is to think about the other party. If you don't, why would you say you are there? Another one is to be a sympathetic audience. Stephen Covey uses this term in Seven Habits of Highly Effective People. Commotional listening implies listening until the other individual feels understood. Sympathetic audience members listen for importance. What are the other individual's thoughts, feelings, and how we can show that we mind substantially?

More than some other relationship appears to forestall development and improvement and makes it harder to accomplish seriousness. It is where one gathering gives a great deal yet receives much less consequently. You wonder whether your partner truly thinks about supporting the relationship.

You truly would prefer not to be associated with relationships that wear you out, exhaust your energy, and aren't responded. Two things differentiate us from our grandparents' age:

- We're more distracted (that isn't very good)
- We're more dedicated to both development and illumination (that is acceptable). The self-awareness industry is developing 6% year over year!

It implies we have more boundaries to conquer concerning growing genuine relationships with genuine individuals. However, it additionally implies we're up for the test.

In general, what would you be able to do to assemble significant relationships? Here are my five hints.

- Make sure you show that your mind about the other individual. Understand their emotions.
- Be mindful of their needs. Come to the situation from their perspective. How might you need them to respond if you had communicated your feelings?
- Be straightforward. Offer your thoughts, thought processes in the relationship, desires. Express lament when you have accomplished something incorrectly and vow not to do it once more.
- Prize yourself and your partner when things work out in a good manner. Offer in the pleasure of the great occasions.
- Notice the main letter of the strong words spells C-A-T-E-R. As such, you have to consider each other's needs to assemble healthy relationships.

Healthy relationships are a two-way road, and both of you should be in a similar place. Continuously ask yourself, what would you be able to improve? You have a confirmed commitment to add importance to your life and the life of your partner. Doing so can be a venturing stone to a more prominent harmony and satisfaction. However, like most things in life, it requires some investment and effort to develop relationships and become the individual we need.

Mindsets for Creating Meaningful Relationships

When it comes to creating meaningful relationships, which is why we go into them, there are two types of mindsets. Out of the two, one is beneficial while the other is destructive. What are these mindsets? Let's look at each of them in detail:

Qualities of Separation Mindset

Here are the normal qualities of somebody with a partition outlook:

- You consider individuals to be discrete with you. They have no relationship to what your identity is.
- You are regularly stressed over the feeling's others have of you.

When meeting another person, you are obsessed with giving the right impression (initial introductions, instead of cultivating a relationship).

You don't open yourself up, nor you completely give your trust to somebody, until he/she has demonstrated deserving it. It is a shield to keep yourself from regularly getting injured.

Thus, you set aside an effort to get ready for individuals before you become calm around them and uncover who you truly are. Before this occurs, you ordinarily venture a front that is very surprising from how you regularly are.

You consider the world a chilly, dim, and risky place with noxious individuals out there to hurt you (or others). E.g., If somebody approaches you in a remote land, your first nature is to wonder if the individual is attempting to pick your pocket or scam you, instead of anything else.

You question individuals' aims (particularly if it's somebody you don't have a clue about), because as your folks consistently say, "You can't be sure whether others have ulterior thought processes." and you like to fail to err on the side of caution.

Issues with Separation Mindset

The division attitude is one that is set apart by fear. It is essentially the wellspring of all issues concerning both social circumstances and relationships. (Note: by relationships, I'm alluding to a wide range of relationships, including fellowships, business relationships, romantic relationships, familial relationships, and so on).

Here are regular issues that somebody with a separation attitude would confront:

- It requires some investment for relationships to manufacture. Rather than getting directly into the core of connecting with individuals immediately, there is regularly a great deal of time spent moving around the edges before becoming more and better acquainted with the individuals. For individuals with deep partition attitudes, it takes significantly more. You make a great deal of superfluous strain for yourself, the other individual, and the other individual in a relationship.
- Within social circumstances, you are frequently worried about whether you're giving the correct

impression instead of concentrating on the communication between you and the other individual.

- You drive away from incredible individuals and extraordinary relationships (be it likely friends or possible romantic partners) without knowing it yourself. That is exactly because you create such huge numbers of insane boundaries for somebody to know you and draw near you, with the end goal, it turns into an inconsequential undertaking for the other party by the day's end.
- You are regularly re-thinking others' expectations instead of assuming the best about them.
- You regularly have issues meeting good individuals, be it friends or romantic partners. For some unknown reasons, you frequently pull in fear-based individuals into your life. That is because of fear-based psychological pulls in fear-based individuals.

Oneness Mindset: Viewing People as Souls to Be Reconnected

Something opposite to the detachment attitude is the oneness outlook. As opposed to considering individuals to be discrete from you, you perceive others as a piece of you, and you are 6 of one, half a dozen of another. It is an attitude set apart by adoration.

Attributes of Oneness Mindset

You consider individuals to be associated with you. Regardless of whether you may not know everybody yet, a relationship as of now exists, and you need to take advantage of that dormant relationship when you meet every individual.

You don't stress yourself with what individuals consider you. You know your expectations are sober, and that is exactly what makes a difference.

Impressions don't concern you. You know the relationship is past the underlying impressions, and it's tied in with building a genuine relationship.

You open up your credible, genuine self when you're around individuals you know, just as individuals you don't have a clue yet. Your heart is worn totally on your sleeve. You don't hole up behind a cover or attempt to be somebody else.

The idea of "warming up" to others doesn't exist. You get right to interfacing with individuals when you (initially) meet them.

You consider the world as one, where everybody is interconnected with one another, uniquely isolated by the space between them. Every individual serves a job in the great structure, and every job the individual serves underpins every other person known to humanity.

Everybody gets the opportunity to be vindicated from you until demonstrated otherwise. You consider everybody to be having real, well-meaning goals in his/her heart, and there is nobody out there attempting to hurt anyone. (A special case to the standard would be individuals in very fear-based cognizance, who have lost their direction and resort to harming others to leave themselves alone hurt.)

Advantages of Oneness Mindset

When you grasp the oneness attitude, you will encounter a significant change in perspective within your social relationships.

There is no fear when you are around individuals since you remember they are pieces of you.

As opposed to investing energy "assembling" the relationship (familiarizing, becoming acquainted with the individual better, knowing the individual's advantages, framing trust, and so on), you get the right to cultivate the relationship immediately.

The idea of time has no importance in the development of your relationship with others. You can be meeting individuals off the bat and turning out to be extraordinary mates with them.

Individuals love to associate with you as a result of the energy you ooze. Simultaneously, you flourish within sight of other magnificent individuals too. There are no boundaries, separators, or separation among you and them.

You have little issue drawing in great, high cognizance individuals into your life. Liberal spirits, kind, holy messengers, strong spirits; these individuals continue to enter your life consistently.

You are a lot more joyful and calm with yourself, contrasted with somebody with a detachment outlook.

You stop stressing over creation great initial introductions and anticipating a specific picture of yourself, rather than taking a shot at fortifying the relationship between you and the other person.

Chapter 10- Better Future with Healthy Relationships

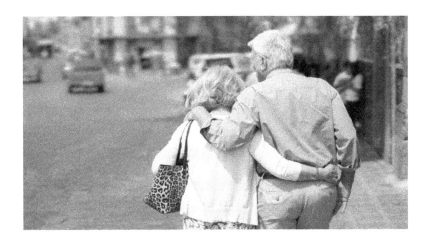

A healthy relationship is a relationship in which the involved parties feel supported, connected, and still feel independent in their way. A healthy relationship equally has the freedom to speak out and voice your concerns without feeling indebted to anyone. When you're in a healthy relationship, you will notice it through your communication and the boundaries you have put.

Signs of a Healthy Relationship

The freedom to speak your mind helps any relationship thrive because it allows couples to express themselves freely and honestly. In such a case, no topic can never be discussed, and this allows both parties to feel they are getting their issues out. Freedom of speech also helps build consistency in a relationship, thus creating a more lasting bond.

Being in love does not mean you need to let go of who you are and spend every single moment with your spouse. You need to have your space to have time to pursue your interests and still keep the relationship or friendship as fresh and exciting as possible. Having your space allows you to grow yourself even as you grow together as a couple.

Whether at work, with your siblings, or a couple, disagreements are unavoidable in any relationship. Disagreements are an ordinary happening despite how much you would like to convince us that you are perfect. If you say you are in a relationship that has no fights, then probably both of you are holding back and are not in your true selves. In a healthy relationship, even disagreements are productive and relatively healthy. That means you will strive by all means to understand your spouse instead of trying to outdo your spouse, and in case you are wrong, you will be willing to apologize.

A healthy relationship is entirely based on reality. You cannot say you do not like someone now than later say you love them. You need to like yourself and your partner just as you are at the present moment. It is not advisable to like someone with the hope that they will change. The freedom that comes as part of a healthy relationship should keep you close, whether he changes or not.

Every relationship has the head, which we often say is the man, but try to make your decisions jointly. Always make it a decision to give an ear to your companion's ideas and, where possible, even give it a try so that nothing is a surprise by the time you rea deciding.

A healthy relationship should be an assured source of joy and laughter. You might not be happy together every other hour of the day because different things happen, but it means that your life together is often delighted. Your partner will once in a while drive up the wall, and you will step on her toe, but because of the love you mutually share, it will not take long before you forgive each other and move on.

It is crucial that in a healthy relationship, there is a balance. You need to find a balance concerning the duties that you are covering. You may need to take care of a sick family member or travel for a business trip. If your relationship is balanced, you will not concentrate on one side but try to find a balance that will make both of you comfortable and happy.

When you can treat the person you love with care and kindness, it makes your relationship adorable and admirable. You might be the kind of people who can feely show respect, appreciation, empathy, and consideration to people who you do not even know, or you are not close more than you do to your partner.

It is essential to trust each other because this is a vital foundation. It is said that broken trust is like broken glass, you might glue the pieces together, but the cracks will never go. You can imagine a broken trust between you and your lover, that doubt will live forever, and trusting each other may be a daydream.

Forgiveness and letting go remain to be an anchor in any relationship. When you can let go of things and smile together, it helps build a bond and create freedom. The freedom created is not to take each other for granted but to understand that we are human beings and are bound to fall. After we fall and have someone remind us, you can rise again without being judgmental; it helps create a real relationship without preteens.

Nothing feels better than the fact you know that you have a relationship that is your fallback plan. You should be with someone you know no matter what happens, you can always come back to them, and you will still be taken in. When you are in such a healthy relationship, you tend to believe that no matter how wrong something is, "I should let know my partner."

Secure your relationship by talking to your partner and not to other people. Sharing your marital issues with your friends and colleges at work might seem to be relieving, but they are not in any position to build your relationship. Your friends will only use your stories to entertain themselves during their breaks and creating a happy hour. Do not use your friends as a crutch to run away from hard conversations with your partner.

Chapter 11- Practical Exercises to Try with Your Partner to Improve Communication

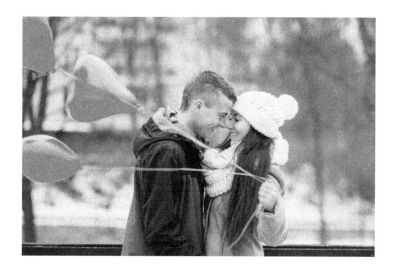

Now that we have spent a lot of time talking about communication and how important it is to your life and your relationship, it is time to look at a few of the practical exercises that you and your partner can use to improve the lines of communication. At this point, you are excited to open up these lines and to get to talking more with your partner than ever before. But you may be unsure of how to put some of the techniques and skills that we have discussed to work.

Communication activities designed for couples are exercises that couples can use to improve how they can converse with one another. As you are working together on these activities, the communication skills will be enhanced, and both partners will learn how to understand one another better. When communication is improved, not only are the words that you speak together butter understood, but the meaning that is behind those words can be understood as well.

There are many communication activities that you can choose to do with your partner. But below, we will talk about some of the most effective methods that will have you and your partner communicating and connecting better than ever before.

Have a Structured Conversation

The first thing that we will look at doing is having a structured conversation with your partner. To make this one work, you need to set aside time to talk with your partner. It needs to be when the two of you can focus just on one another, and there are no distractions. Turn the phones off, put the computer down, and ensure that the kids are in bed or over with the babysitter (grandma can work too).

Then, you need to discuss some topics that the two of you want to talk about. Once this topic is selected, both partners need to begin talking. But instead of communicating as you normally do, you need to add a bit more structure to the mix. You can add this to the dialog by using empathy, validation, and mirroring. Mirroring is when you repeat what your partner said but express that you are interested and curious in your own words.

Validating is another tool that you can use. It is when you are going to show your partner that you understand what they are saying. Often, the only thing you need to say for this one is "I get what you're saying" or something similar. And finally, you need to show some empathy in the conversation as well. This empathy expresses interest in how your partner feels by saying something and asking questions to get to the bottom of things and try and understand them.

When you and your partner take the time to sit down and do some structured conversation, you are making sure that you get a chance to be alone and focus on each other. You pay attention to the other person so that you can mirror them, validate them, and empathize with them. And you will be surprised at how this simple little thing can open them up to you and can make them more receptive to the things that you tell them as well.

Play Positive Language Games

The next exercise to work on is playing positive language games. For this one, both partners in the relationship need to replace any negative language that they use with something more positive. If you stop and think carefully about it, we all use way too much negative language in our lives. We often do this on autopilot, without even thinking about it. But the subconscious of the other person in the relationship will catch on to information, and they will catch the negative things that are said.

Even if we don't mean to talk with negative language, we are bringing the other person down. They are going to feel bad and may start to feel a bit of resentment towards you. It can close them down to any form of communication with you because they don't want to feel negative any longer. Often, both partners are going to do this to some degree. It is why we need to focus on improving our language and change it from negative over to positive.

So, to make this one work, the next time you feel that you will say something negative about your partner about something that they have said or done, stop and find a new, more positive way that you can get your message out there to your partner.

When you stop and do this kind of exercise, it forces you to become more aware of the different ways you communicate with your partner, and you may start to notice that you are communicating negatively with them. You can then reverse some of your negative communication patterns and start saying more positive things.

The good news is that most partners have no want to come across as judgmental and accusatory to the person they love. They don't realize that they are coming across as so negative in the process. When you use this exercise and play positive love games, you can start to see how you talk to your partner, even if you don't mean to do it this way, and you can make the necessary changes.

Go on A Trip Together

This one may sound surprising, but planning and going on a trip with your partner can be a great therapy exercise for improving your communication. This trip means that you and your partner will get at least one day, but usually more, alone in a new and exciting environment.

The reason that is going on a trip together can be such an effective therapy because it allows the couples to unwind, get away from all the hustle and bustle that comes with their daily lives, and gives them a chance to relax. And when you can get away, you will find that it can do wonders for improving communication.

It is amazing what can happen when you can take the stress out of your life. Communicating with anyone, even your partner, when you are stressed out and tired is going to be hard. And many of the disagreements and misunderstandings you go through with your partner are because one or both of you are stressed out and tired.

If you would like to build up the amount of communication that is in your relationship, you must take the time to promote stress relief as much as possible. When the stress is gone, it allows you and your partner to focus on each other while you converse and connect on a deeper level. Even the planning part can be helpful here because you both need to communicate effectively to get all of the plans in order.

If you have kids, it is especially important to find some time away from them, and maybe go on a small trip without them. While it is always fun to take the kids on vacation with you, there isn't going to be a lot of deep and meaningful communication between you and your partner. Most of the conversation will be with your children and the logistics of taking care of them. There is nothing wrong with taking your kids on vacation, but it is fine for you and your partner to go off on your own for a bit every once in a while. Even if it is just a weekend to the nearest city for a hotel stay, it still gives you a chance to plan out something together and spend together without others.

Conclusion

This book has been a great read for those struggling in their relationships or looking to improve their communication skills. Communication is an important part of any relationship, and you and your partner need to be able to communicate about things that matter.

Communication is a lost art in today's society. To build a strong and healthy relationship, you should be able to speak openly about all aspects of your life. Communication is so important, and it's important to talk about things that are going on in your relationship. Keeping things bottled up can lead to problems in the relationship itself, and you should always be able to express yourself.

This last guide will summarize what you have learned in this ultimate guide so that you can be a more successful couple. If you have a strong relationship, then you're on your way to success.

Both of you need to understand each other's feelings, needs, wants, and desires. The easiest way for this to occur or happen is by being honest with each other throughout the whole process. Honesty is the best policy, and it's important to never lie to your partner. Honesty is very important to any relationship, and you should always express your thoughts and feelings.

Honesty is also important for communication because it is the foundation of any relationship. If you aren't honest with each other, then how can you expect a healthy relationship? You must be honest to have a happy relationship.

You should always try to understand each other's point of view. It is essential, and you should always be open-minded and willing to listen to what your partner has to say. Both of you need to know what the other person wants out of the relationship, which will help improve your communication if you both understand each other.

You must communicate with each other for things to go well in your relationship. When communication is going well, it will lead to a stronger bond. If you understand each other's feelings, then you'll be able to have many conversations with each other.

It's also important for both of you to understand the other person's needs. If you don't understand your partner's needs, then they will become frustrated and become angry with you over little things. You need to be aware of your partner's needs to help them feel better and have a good relationship.

You should always try and have conflict resolution discussions with your partner. You need to resolve things quickly to avoid conflict, which doesn't have to happen simultaneously. Conflict is very common, but you should always handle a situation calmly and professionally. Being able to resolve things calmly is important because it will give both of you a good thought process and will make you a better couple overall.

Silence is not the solution for the conflict. If you're angry at your partner, then you should express those feelings. Both of you need to be able to communicate how you feel through conflict. It will help reduce the tension in the relationship, and both of you can come to a resolution that suits everyone.

You need to understand that conflict is also very common in relationships. Communication is how you resolve things in this situation, and both of you need to be able to talk about occurring problems. If you can't talk about it, you should try and work through it.

You need to try and solve problems calmly. If you don't know how to solve a problem, then resolution through communication is the best way to go about it. You should always resolve issues in your relationship. Still, if you aren't going to have a conversation with your partner, you shouldn't expect that they will understand what is going on in your relationship otherwise.

If you want to improve your relationship, then you should have communication with each other. Communication is the way to build a close bond as a couple, and neither of you should be afraid to express your feelings. You must always communicate with each other to go well, which will make both of you happy. Communication is an essential pillar of any relationship, and both partners in the relationship need to understand and express their feelings throughout the whole process.

Finally, we hope that this book has helped you improve your relationships and help you have a good relationship with your partner. Good luck with your effective communication, and we hope for good things to come to your relationship.

CPSIA information can be obtained
at www.ICGtesting.com
Printed in the USA
BVHW041517190321
602997BV00010B/596